BEI GRIN MACHT SICH IHR WISSEN BEZAHLT

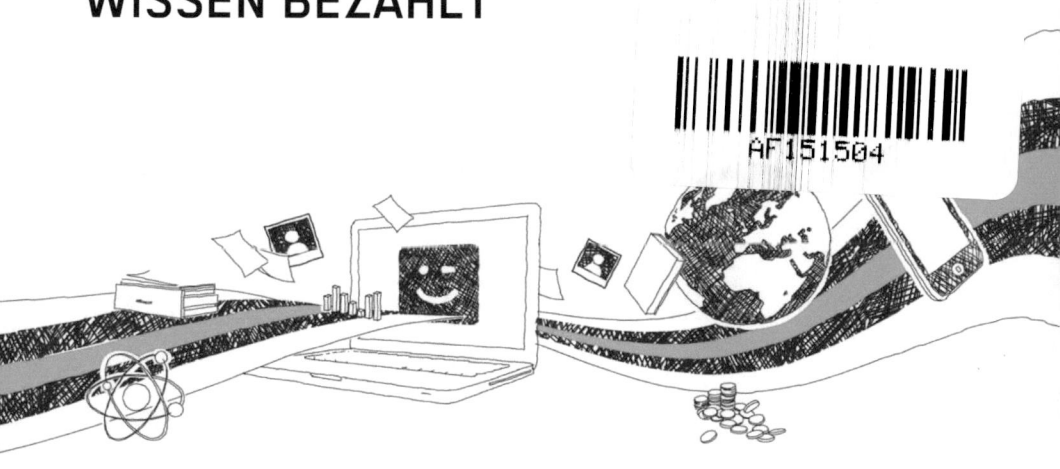

- Wir veröffentlichen Ihre Hausarbeit, Bachelor- und Masterarbeit

- Ihr eigenes eBook und Buch - weltweit in allen wichtigen Shops

- Verdienen Sie an jedem Verkauf

Jetzt bei www.GRIN.com hochladen und kostenlos publizieren

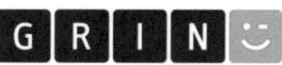

Peter Ubah Okeke

Women Use of Oral Contraceptives - Does it have any Effect on Haematological Parameters?

GRIN Verlag

Bibliografische Information der Deutschen Nationalbibliothek:

Die Deutsche Bibliothek verzeichnet diese Publikation in der Deutschen National-
bibliografie; detaillierte bibliografische Daten sind im Internet über http://dnb.d-
nb.de/ abrufbar.

Impressum:

Copyright © 2011 GRIN Verlag GmbH
Druck und Bindung: Books on Demand GmbH, Norderstedt Germany
ISBN: 978-3-640-97697-3

Dieses Buch bei GRIN:

http://www.grin.com/de/e-book/176326/women-use-of-oral-contraceptives-does-
it-have-any-effect-on-haematological

WOMEN USE OF ORAL CONTRACEPTIVES, DOES IT HAVE ANY EFFECT ON HAEMATOLOGICAL PARAMETERS ?

BY

PETER UBAH OKEKE

CAPE VERDE, 2011

AIMS AND OBJECTIVES: **To study the effect of oral contraceptives on haematological parameters of Hemoglobin, Hematocrit, Red blood cell count, White blood cell count, Mean cell volume, Mean cell Hemoglobin, Mean cell Hemoglobin concentration, Platelet count and Red cell distribution width- Coefficient variation in apparently healthy women of Porto Novo.**

KEYWORDS: **Blood count, oral contraceptives, women.**

CORRESPONDING AUTHOR: **Peter Ubah Okeke; Medical Technologist, Dept. of Medical laboratory Science, Hospital of Porto Novo- Cape Verde.**

ABSTRACT

The results of 90 apparently healthy women between the age of 17 to 39 years old on oral contraceptives for not less than six months tested for hematological parameters for the month of July, 2011and comparing the results obtained with the local reference values showed that ;Rbc: 4.40 × $10^{9/L}$, Hb:12.38g/dl, Ht: 38.1L/L, MCV:86.94FL, MCH:28.8pg, MCHC:31.50 %, RDW-CV: 12.98, Total WBC:7.40× $10^{9/L}$, Platelet 272× $10^{9/L}$ all values in mean were recorded. It was observed that 1.1% were thrombocytopenic and anemic, whereas 3.3% were of the mild leucocytosis. Nevertheless, the results were not clinical and statistical significant.

Finally the study concluded that no significant effects were observed on hematological parameters due to oral contraceptive use and the women of Porto Novo should continue to use oral contraceptives correctly to prevent unwanted and or unnecessary pregnancies with the instruction of a Nursing officer in charge of the reproductive section.

Introduction

Combination contraceptives are most effective means for contraception excluding sterilization. Contraceptives are hormonal agents, combination oral contraceptives contain both an estrogen and a progestogen. Endogenous estrogens are largely responsible for the development and maintenance of female reproductive system and secondary sexual characteristics. Estrogens act through binding to nuclear receptors in estrogen responsive tissues

Circulating estrogens modulate the pituitary secretion of the gonadotropins, luteinizing hormone(LH) and follicle stimulating hormone (FSH), through a negative feedback mechanism. Modern progestogens such as gestodene have been developed in order to provide women with an oral contraceptive agent with more selective progestational activity that improves cycle control, minimizes metabolic changes and adverse events and effectively prevents pregnancy.

Of these agents, gestodene has been shown to be a particularly effective inhibitor of ovarian activity with a pronounced progestational effect on the endometrium in both preclinical and clinical trials, Gast MJ (1996). Gestodene has been combined with low doses of ethinylestradiol to provide low- dose combination oral contraceptive preparations. While low dose combination oral contraceptives are the most widely prescribed form of oral contraceptive today and have a low failure rate in terms of unintended pregnancies, Aguiar et al (1996) reported that approximately 50% of all women who begins taking oral contraceptives discontinue their use within one year. Of the factors attributed to non-compliance and or discontinuation of it according to Aguiar and co-workers, include, poor cycle control, amenorrhea, headache, weight gain and breast tenderness.

Dr. Heli Bathija(1998) reported higher hemoglobin and Ferritin levels on women taking oral contraceptives and concluded that hemoglobin and Ferritin levels are influenced by the use of contraceptives and that the hormonal contraceptives included in his studies have a beneficial effects on these parameters.

Professor Vessey M P (1993) wrote that oral contraceptives offer protection against both epithelial cancer of the ovary and cancer of the endometrium and protection increases with duration of use and persists for at least 15 years after stopping its use. According to Professor Vessey, well established risks of combined oral contraceptives are mainly vascular ones, comprising effects on acute myocardial infarction, thrombotic stroke, haemorrhagic stroke and venous thrombosis and embolism.

Dr. Brown and co-workers (1988) expressed that oral contraceptives protects against menstrual bleeding problems and thereby reduce the risk of iron- deficiency anaemia. They also afford protection against benign breast disease Brinton L.A. et al (1981).

Mooij PN et al (1992) reported no significant difference on hematological parameters due to oral contraceptive use in women but serum iron status were significantly increased for the users of oral contraceptive. According to Charles JP et al (1975), serum folate levels were not significantly affected and there were no macrocytosis and no hypersegemented polymorphonuclear leucocytes among the users of oral contraceptives. This shows that oral contraceptive agents do not cause folate deficiency anaemia in otherwise normal subjects.

The experiment of Irwin Fisch & Shanna Freedman (1975) demonstrated that red blood cells variables were lesser significant in women that are taking oral contraceptives, however total leucocyte count were slightly raised.

Dr. Burton J L(1967) reported that serum iron and serum total iron binding capacity were strikingly elevated in women taken oral contraceptives and this was attributed in part to a response to circulating oestrogens and or progesterone. Dr. Godsland et al (1983) investigated haematological indices and metabolic effects of oral contraceptives and concluded that no statistically significant effects were observed. England & Bain BJ (1976) reported that some form of oral contraceptives raise the leucocyte count.

In this study, the aim was to investigate the effect of oral contraceptives on some haematological parameters of Red blood cell count, Haemoglobin, Haematocrit, Total white cell count, Platelet count, Mean cell volume (MCV), Mean cell haemoglobin (MCH), Mean cell haemoglobin concentration (MCHC) and Red cell distribution width in coefficient variation, comparing all the values obtained from the women on oral contraceptives with the local reference values.

MATERIALS AND METHODS

 A total of ninety (90) blood samples of apparently healthy women on oral contraceptives for at least six months were collected into K_2EDTA anticoagulant tubes with duration of blood collection of a month (from 1-07-2011 to 31-07-2011). Haematological parameters testing were done using sysmex KX-21-N produced by sysmex corporation Japan , all testing were done at the laboratory science section of the Hospital -Porto Novo.

The hematological parameters of 90 apparently healthy women on oral contraceptives for not less than six months were tested in the Medical laboratory section of the Hospital of Porto Novo and the results were (mean values) as follows: Red blood cell count;$4.40 \times 10^{9/L}$, Hemoglobin; 12.4g/dl, Hematocrit;38.2L/L, Mean Cell Volume;86.9FL, Mean Cell Hemoglobin;28.8Pg, Mean Cell Hemoglobin Concentration; 31.5%, Red Cell Distribution-coefficient variation;12.98%, Total White Cell count;$7.40 \times 10^{9/L}$, Platelet count;$272 \times 10^{9/L}$

Key: Reference values of Porto Novo Laboratory were;Rbc;$4.5 \times 10^{9/L}$, Hb;12.5g/dl, Ht,36%, MCV; 80-100fl, MCH;27-33pg, MCHC;32-36%, WBC;$4-10 \times 10^{9/L}$, RDW-CV;12.8%, Platelet;$150-450 \times 10^{9/L}$

The table below presents the results;

Table 1:Presents hematological parameters (mean) of apparently healthy women on oral contraceptives in Porto Novo, July, 2011(n=90).

HEMATOLOGY PARAMATERS n:90	RBC× $10^{9/L}$	Hb× $10^{9/L}$	Hct $^{L/L}$	MCV FL	MCH Pg	MCHC g/dl	RDW-CV %	WBC× $10^{9/L}$	PLT × $10^{9/L}$
MEAN (π)	4.40	12.4	38	86.9	28.8	31.5	12.9	7.40	272

Table 2: Presents hematological parameters of the 90 apparently healthy women on oral contraceptives in Porto Novo July 2011, mean according to the age group.

HEMATOLOGY PARAMETERS AGE IN YEARS	NUMBER n	RBC× $10^{9/L}$	Hb× $10^{9/L}$	Hct $^{L/L}$	MCV FL	MCH Pg	MCHC g/dl	RDW-CV %	WBC× $10^{9/L}$	PLT × $10^{9/L}$
17-22	33	4.41	12.52	38.8	88.28	27.58	32.26	13.05	6.87	294
23-28	35	4.47	13.17	39.3	88.0	28.8	32.69	12.94	7.06	261
29-39	22	4.31	12.63	39.0	58.11	29.4	32.62	12.94	6.65	258

DISCUSSION AND CONCLUSION

The hematological parameters of ninety (90) apparently healthy women on oral contraceptives were determined, comparing their values with that of the local reference value of the people of Porto Novo and the results were as follows; Rbc ;4.40 $\times 10^{9/L}$, Hb; 12.4g/dl, Ht;38.2L/L, MCV;86.94FL, MCH;28.8Pg, MCHC;31.5%, RDW-CV;12.98%, White cell count;7.40 $\times 10^{9/L}$, and Platelet count;272 $\times 10^{9/L}$.

The effect of 1.1% of thrombocytopenia, 1.1% of anemia and 3.3% mild leucocytosis were observed but not clinical and statistical significant. This work agreed in part with that of Mooij PN et al(1992) who reported no clinical and statistical significant of hematological parameters of women on oral contraceptives but the parameters of serum iron were elevated to a significant degree, although the parameters tested in this work do not include serum iron estimation. The results based on the age of the women did not show any definite pattern but also were normal within the local reference interval of the population.

Dr. Heli Bathija(1998) observed higher hemoglobin values and ferritin levels on women taking oral contraceptives than those who do not take, this is beneficial in reducing anemic incidence within these women.

Professor M. P. Vessey(1993) summarized that oral contraceptives protects against iron deficiency anemia and protection increases with duration of use. The results obtained here also showed that the women using oral pills, used it correctly and this could protect them from excessive menstrual blood loss.

The Porto Novo studies also agreed with Dr. Godsland et al (1983) who reported no significant differences observed on studying hematological indices of women taking oral contraceptives.

The leucocyte count observed in this study were within normal in contrast with that of England et al (1976) who stated raised leucocyte count among women on oral contraceptives.

The results obtained could have been influenced by the modern pharmaceutical preparation of the oral contraceptives with the diminution of the added materials thereby reducing to the minimum its effect on blood cells.

The conclusion was that no significant hematological effect were seen on women taking oral contraceptives and the women of Porto Novo municipality should continue to use the pills to prevent unnecessary or unwanted pregnancies but with the orientation of the nurse in charge of the reproductive section.

REFERENCES

Aguiar LF et al (1996); Monophasic gestodene and ethinylestradiol in oral contraception: a multicenter open study. Gynecol Endocrinol (10):21-26.

Brinton LA et al (1981); Risk factors for benign breast disease. Am. J Epidemiol (113):203- 14.

Brown S et al (1988); The influence of method of contraception and cigarette smoking on menstrual patterns. Br. J. Obstet Gynecol (92):905-10.

Burton JL(1967); Effect of oral contraceptives on Hb, Pcv, serum iron and TIBC in healthy women. Lancet(289):978-980.

Charles J Paine et al (1975); Oral contraceptives, serum folate and hematological status. Jama 231:731-733.

Collins DC (1994); Sex hormone receptor binding, progestin selectivity and the new oral contraceptives. Am. J. obstetric Gynecol(170). 1508.

Cruickshank JM et al (1970); The effect of age, parity, haemoglobin level and oral contraceptive preparations on the normal leucocyte count. British J. Haematology 18:541.

Dacie & Lewis(2006); Practical Haematology tenth edn. Pg 20-21.

Dodsworth H et al (1981); Effects of smoking and the pill on the blood count. British J. Haematology 49(3):484-8.

Dr. Heli Bathija (1998); Effects of contraceptives on hemoglobin and Ferritin. Contraception vol.58 (5),11:261-273.

England JM et al (1976); Total and differential count. British J. haematology(33):1-7.

Gast MJ(1996); A new generation of oral contraceptive progestins. Gynecol Endocinol(10):1-3.

Godsland et al (1983); Comparison of haematological indices between women of four ethnic groups and the effect of oral contraceptives. J. clinical pathology(36):184-191.

Irwin R. Fisch & Shanna H. Freedman (1975); Smoking, Oral contraceptives and obesity, Effects on white cell count. Jama 234:500-506.

Mooij PN et al (1992); The effects of oral contraceptives and multivitamin supplementation on serum Ferritin and hematological parameters. Int J Pharmacol Ther Toxicol.30(2):57-62.

Rossmanith WG et al; A comparative randomized trial on the impact of two low- dose oral contraceptives on ovarian activity, cervical permability and endometrial receptivity. Contraception 56:23-30.

Sartoretto JN(1977); Clinical studies with a low dose estrogen-progestogen combination. Contraception 15:563-570.

Vessy M P (1993); Benefits and risks of combined oral contraceptives. Methods of information in medicine,32:222-4.

Wild MI & Balfour JA (1995); Gestodene: A review of its pharmacology, efficacy and tolerability in combined contraceptive preparations. Drugs (50): 364-395.